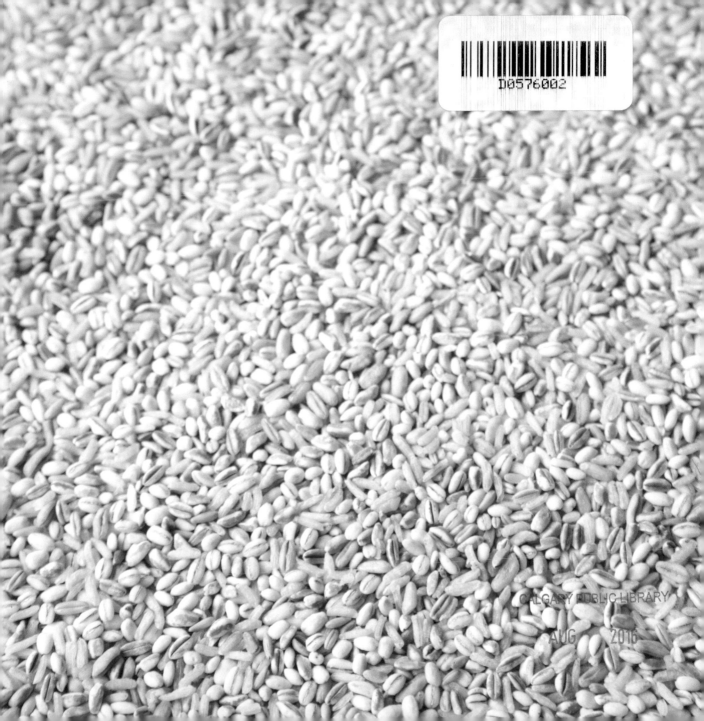

POWER GRAINS

SPELT, FARRO, FREEKEH, AMARANTH, KAMUT, QUINOA AND OTHER ANCIENT GRAINS

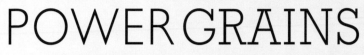

POWER GRAINS

SPELT, FARRO, FREEKEH, AMARANTH, KAMUT, QUINOA AND OTHER ANCIENT GRAINS

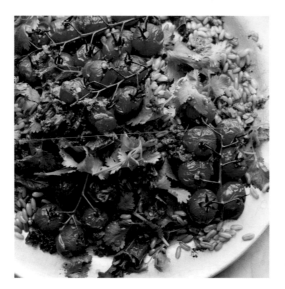

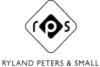

RYLAND PETERS & SMALL
LONDON • NEW YORK

Senior Designer Sonya Nathoo
Commissioning Editor Stephanie Milner
Picture Manager Christina Borsi
Production Manager David Hearn
Art Director Leslie Harrington
Editorial Director Julia Charles
Publisher Cindy Richards

Indexer Hilary Bird

First published in 2016 by Ryland Peters & Small
20–21 Jockey's Fields, London WC1R 4BW and
341 E 116th St, New York, NY 10029
www.rylandpeters.com

10 9 8 7 6 5 4 3 2 1

Design and photographs © Ryland Peters
& Small 2016

ISBN: 978-1-84975-721-8

Printed in China

A CIP record for this book is available from the British Library. US
Library of Congress cataloging-in-publication data has been applied for.

Notes:

• Both British (Metric) and American (Imperial plus US cups)
measurements are included in these recipes for your convenience;
however, it is important to work with one set of measurements and not
alternate between the two within a recipe.

• All spoon measurements are level unless otherwise specified.

• All eggs are medium (UK) or large (US), unless specified as large,
in which case US extra-large should be used. Uncooked or partially
cooked eggs should not be served to the very old, frail, young children,
pregnant women or those with compromised immune systems.

• Ovens should be preheated to the specified temperatures. We
recommend using an oven thermometer. If using a fan-assisted oven,
adjust temperatures according to the manufacturer's instructions.

• When a recipe calls for the grated zest of citrus fruit, buy unwaxed fruit
and wash well before using.

CONTENTS

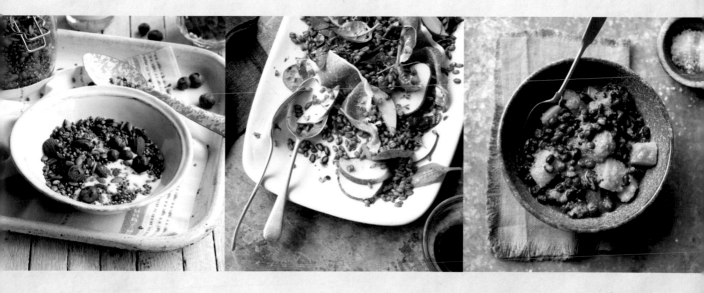

introduction

Grains have been the most important staple foods in just about every corner of the globe since man first grew and harvested crops. They are nutritious and delicious and can be cooked in hundreds of different and exciting ways to create healthy, satisfying meals. In recent years, more and more interesting and unusual varieties have become available and these make a great addition to any modern cook's repertoire. Wholegrains are an essential part of a healthy diet and a great source of complex carbohydrates, fibre/fiber, vitamins and minerals. Even better is that they have the nutrition and taste to stand alone as a meal.

As our desire to try new flavours and embrace ideas from cultures other than our own grows, we learn more about the incredible range of ways in which these foods can be prepared and enjoyed.

The recipes in this book have been culled from different styles of cooking from around the world and all feature grains as their main ingredient, or sometimes a combination of more than one.

Cooking grains can seem intimidating, but they are more forgiving than we think. To simplify, there are two general ways to cook grains. One is the 'absorption' method, where grains are cooked slowly in a specific amount of liquid until tender. Use this for quinoa, millet, amaranth and bulgur. The other way is the 'pasta' method, where grains are cooked in an abundance of water and then drained once cooked, which is better for firmer grains, including barley, buckwheat, farro and wheatberries. For the more experienced chef, there is also the 'toast absorption' method – a variation of the 'absorption' method – where you toast the grains before the liquid is added to increase the amount of flavour in a dish. Each of the recipes in this book indicates which cooking method is best for the dish, but it's good to keep these basic rules in mind should you want to experiment with other combinations of ingredients.

Some grains can be soaked or dry-roasted before cooking, but it's not essential. Soaking hard grains (barley, spelt and so on) makes them easier to digest, as does cooking them in a pressure cooker. Dry-roasting results in an enhanced nutty flavour. Adding soft grains (millet, amaranth, quinoa, etc.) to boiling water cooks them evenly and reduces stickiness.

Grains should be rinsed (if not pre-rinsed) and stored in sterilized airtight containers in the cupboard. It's best to store flours made from grains in the fridge to prolong their shelf life. Grains stay fresh for up to 3 days in the refrigerator once cooked, but they can also be frozen. Some grains freeze better than others and most gluten-free (GF) grains are best eaten fresh. Any gluten-free grains used in soups are also suitable to freeze. Grains and legumes, if cooked on their own, will keep in the refrigerator for 2–4 days.

Gluten is a protein commonly found in wheat and wheat-related species. Many wholegrains also contain this protein, but if you do not have an issue with gluten, then these grains are wonderful additions to your diet. Whether you are a coeliac, gluten sensitive, or have someone you cook for that is, knowing which grains are gluten-free is very important. Many of these grains, like quinoa, millet and amaranth, are related to plant and grass species, rather than wheat, making them gluten-free. These gluten-free grains can be used in their flour form as well, which is convenient for the gluten-free baker, but be sure to check the packet first.

Use these recipes to create healthy and balanced meals. Don't be afraid to experiment and create your own favourites, too!

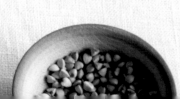

power grain glossary

This book focuses on wholegrains, along with fruits, vegetables, healthy fats and protein. Each grain has certain nutritional value, outlined below.

Amaranth (GF)
This gluten-free grass species was cultivated by Aztecs and Incas, and has a similar nutritional value to quinoa. High in protein, calcium, potassium, magnesium and folic acid, it's a grain that is definitely worth trying. A small ancient grain, amaranth retains a little texture once cooked.

Barley
A high-fibre/fiber, nutty-flavoured grain most commonly used in soups. It is sold in many forms, depending on how much of the outer covering is removed. Hulled barley, with the bran layer still intact, but the outermost layer removed, retains the nutrition from the bran layer but needs cooking for longer than other barleys as well as soaking the night before. Pearl barley is most commonly available – an underrated and economical alternative to rice, with its soft, slightly nutty grain – and cooks more quickly than barley, as it has had its outer bran and husk removed.

Buckwheat (GF)
Completely wheat- and gluten-free, buckwheat contains all the essential amino acids: calcium, potassium, iron and zinc; has a low glycemic index (GI), is high in protein, and rich in magnesium, which we could all do with more of. You can buy the kernels (groats) in bulk, or buckwheat flour to use in healthy baking recipes. It has received a lot of attention recently for its apparent ability to lower blood sugar levels, which would be great news for diabetics.

Bulgur
A common Middle Eastern grain, this cracked wheat is high in fibre/fiber, low in calories and quick to cook. It is traditionally used in tabbouleh but can be made into any cold grain salad.

Farro
These whole-wheat kernels are sweet, chewy and nutty, and high in fibre/fiber, magnesium and vitamins A, E and B. They are common in Tuscan cooking and great in salads and soups.

Freekeh
A young-harvested wheat, this grain is smoky to taste and high in fibre/fiber and protein. Because of this, it is commonly used in salads and side dishes.

Kamut
With a higher percentage of lipids (naturally occurring fats and oils) than other grains, kamut is a good energy source. It is larger than other grains so can hold its own in dishes like pilafs.

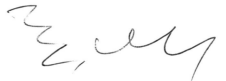

Millet (GF)

Best served hot, this gluten-free grain is a good alternative to couscous, while the flour, which is now commonly sold in health-food markets, can be used for baking. Millet is high in nutrients such as magnesium and manganese.

Oats

The low GI of oats supports well-being by slowly raising blood sugar for energy, while the soluble fibre/fiber content reduces cholesterol. Use organic oats if you can. Oats are naturally gluten-free but many brands process them in factories that process wheat. Oats processed in wheat-free factories should be labelled 'gluten-free'.

Quinoa (GF)

A complete food that contains all the essential amino acids, is high in protein, iron, potassium and phosphorous, and is easily digestible. Quinoa, although technically a grass species, has similar power-giving properties to other grains and is very versatile – you can have it sweet, savoury, cold, hot, and it tastes good leftover, too. The most common colours are white and red, although it is also available in black or purple. Quinoa is a fantastic source of easily digested protein – 200 g/1 cup quinoa provides 3 g more protein than an egg!

Spelt

This nutrient powerhouse has a high water solubility so nutrients from other ingredients are easily absorbed. It is also high in fibre/fiber. Those with mild gluten sensitivity often tolerate the gluten found in spelt. Spelt flour is great to bake with for those who can tolerate gluten. It is technically an ancient form of wheat, but it is easier to digest than standard wheat, higher in protein and the B-complex vitamins.

Teff (GF)

Teff is the smallest of the gluten-free grains, but it is not small in nutritional value. Higher in calcium and vitamin C than any other grain, teff is best used as a flour in baked goods. It comes from Ethiopia, where they use it to bake bread called *injera*.

Other healthy ingredients

'Superfood' is a bit of a catchy word used to describe foods that are exceptional in nutritional value. Many of the wholegrains used in this book are superfoods, but there are a few other foods worth noting. These include omega-3-rich flax, chia and hemp seeds, antioxidant pumpkin seeds and coconut oil with its medium-chain fatty acids. Berries and sprouted vegetables are excellent, too. All are a healthy addition to any diet; high in antioxidants, rich in fibre/fiber and packed full of potassium – super!

BREAKFASTS

This is a very hearty and satisfying breakfast or the perfect pre-exercise boost. You can use any nut butter that you have to hand – try almond or cashew butter for a paleo smoothie.

peanut butter oat shake

35 g/⅓ cup gluten-free rolled oats
360 ml/1½ cups almond milk
1 banana
4 tablespoons peanut butter
2 tablespoons agave syrup
170 g/1 cup ice cubes

SERVES 2

Pour the almond milk over the oats; cover and chill in the fridge for 20 minutes, until the oats are soft.

When the oats are ready, put the almond-soaked oats, banana, peanut butter, agave syrup and ice in a food processor and blend to a smooth consistency. Serve immediately.

The perfect on-the-go breakfast, this purple-coloured smoothie is packed full of health-giving antioxidants and high-energy oats, and tastes just as good as it looks!

blueberry oat smoothie

35 g/⅓ cup gluten-free rolled oats
360 ml/1½ cups almond milk
130 g/1 cup frozen blueberries or mixed berries
120 g/½ cup plain yogurt
2 tablespoons honey
75 g/⅓ cup ice cubes

SERVES 2

Pour the almond milk over the oats; cover and chill in the fridge for 20 minutes, until the oats are soft.

When the oats are ready, put the almond-soaked oats, blueberries, yogurt, honey and ice in a food processor and blend to a smooth consistency. Serve immediately.

The texture of oats in a morning muffin feels very hearty. Oat flour is a great alternative to plain/all-purpose flour and works really well as a substitution for other flours in baked goods, as well as providing a boost of energy from power grains.

fruit and oat muffins

100 g/1 cup (gluten-free) rolled oats
90 g/²⁄₃ cup (gluten-free) oat flour
100 g/³⁄₄ cup plain/all-purpose flour
   (plus ½ teaspoon xanthan gum
   if using gluten-free plain/
   all-purpose flour)
110 g/½ cup brown sugar
1 teaspoon baking powder
1 teaspoon bicarbonate of/
   baking soda
½ teaspoon salt
2 eggs
1 teaspoon pure vanilla extract
100 ml/⅓ cup vegetable oil
100 g/1 cup fresh or frozen mixed
   berries
milk, to serve (optional)

Fruit purée
150 ml/²⁄₃ cup soy milk
about 5 dried figs
80 g/⅓ cup pineapple pieces

a 12-hole muffin pan, greased

MAKES 12

Begin by making the fruit purée. Put 60 ml/¼ cup of warm water, the soy milk, figs and pineapple in a food processor and blend to a thick consistency. Set aside.

Preheat the oven to 180°C (350°F) Gas 4.

Mix together the oats, flours, sugar, baking powder, bicarbonate of/baking soda and salt in a large mixing bowl. In a separate bowl, mix together the prepared fruit purée, eggs, xanthan gum (if using), vanilla and oil. Add the dry mixture into the wet a little at a time before folding in the mixed berries.

Pour the batter into the prepared muffin pan and bake in the preheated oven for 20 minutes, or until a knife inserted into the middle comes out clean. Remove from the oven and set aside to cool before serving with a glass of milk for a childhood treat.

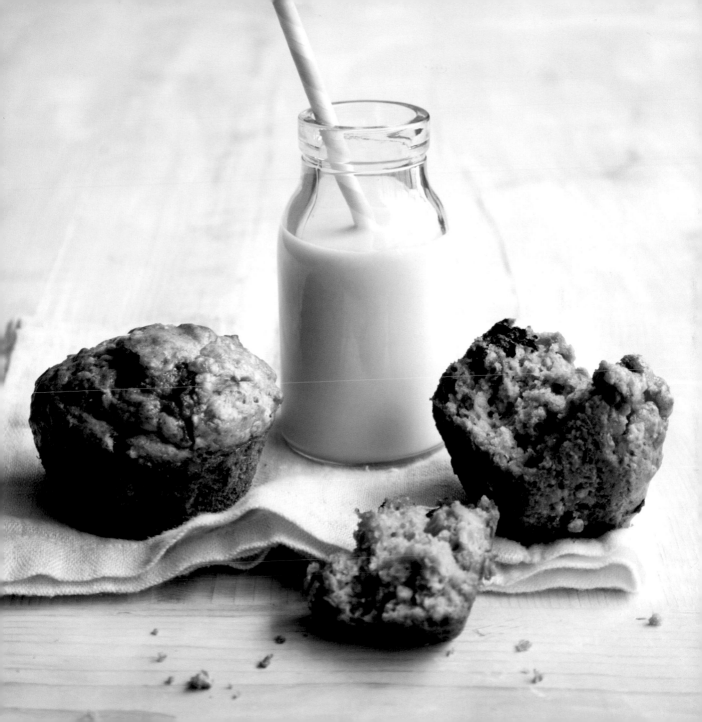

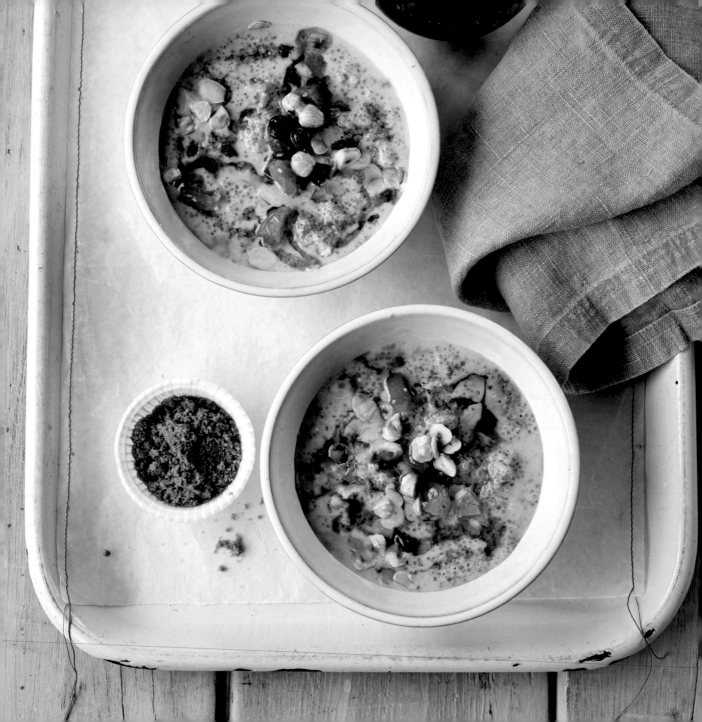

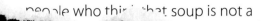

people who think that soup is not a

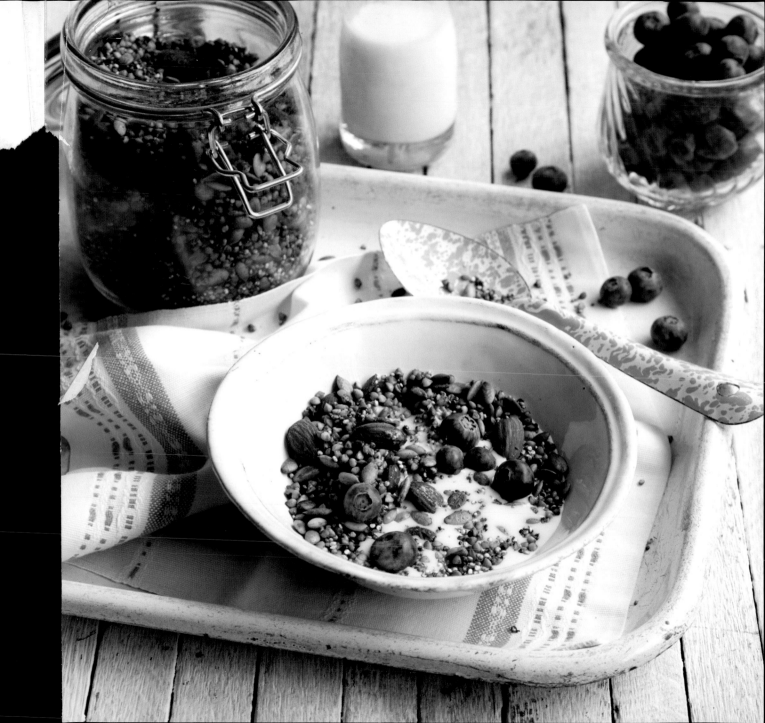

SOUPS AND SALADS

QUINOA · VEGAN · GLUTEN-FREE · DAIRY-FREE

This is a great take on

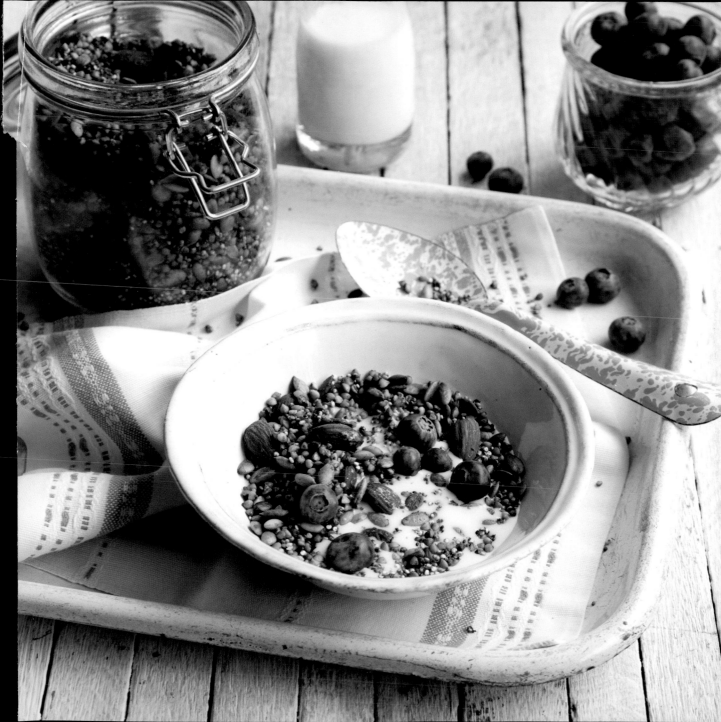

SOUPS AND SALADS

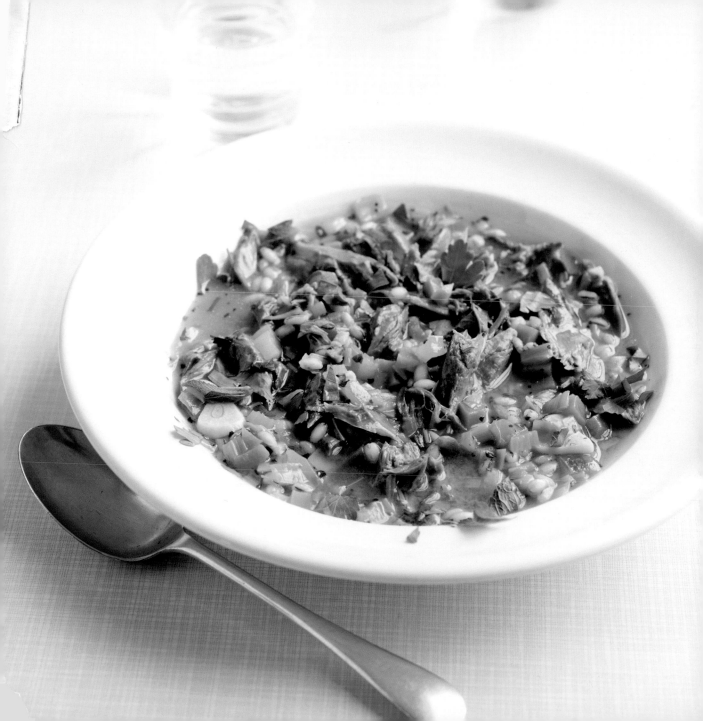

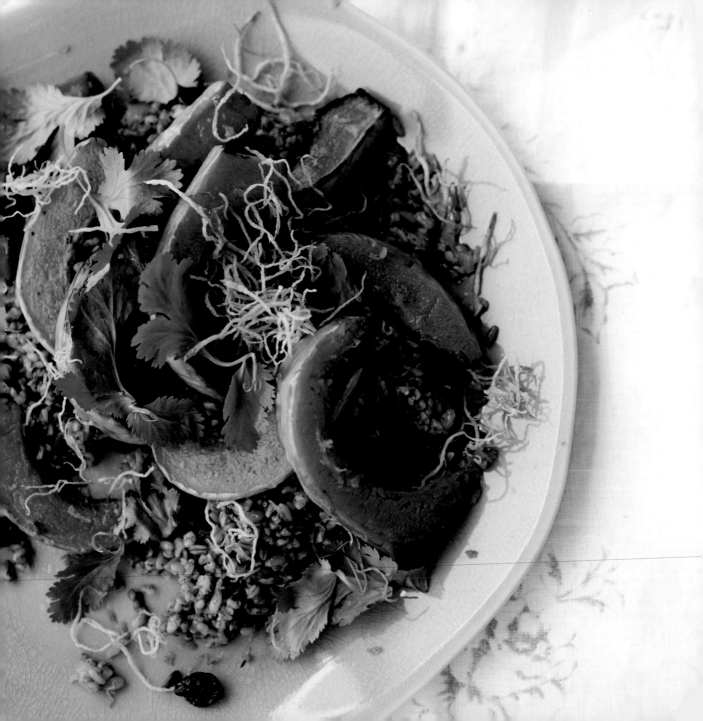

Like quinoa, freekeh is rich in protein and has a slightly nutty, earthy taste, but you can use quinoa instead, or even bulgur wheat. Middle Eastern in origin, freekeh is a green wheat that is picked unripe and then roasted to give it a slight smokiness.

freekeh, pumpkin and crispy ginger salad

500 g/1 lb 2 oz. pumpkin or butternut squash, skin removed, seeded and cut into pieces
3 tablespoons olive oil
125 g/1 cup freekeh
3-cm/1¼-in. piece fresh root ginger, peeled and cut into thin strips
1 large onion, chopped
2 large garlic cloves, chopped
3 handfuls of sultanas/golden raisins
finely grated zest and freshly squeezed juice of 1 orange
1 teaspoon ground allspice
1 teaspoon ground ginger
a squeeze of lemon juice
2 handfuls of freshly chopped coriander/cilantro leaves, plus a few whole leaves to decorate
sea salt and freshly ground black pepper, to taste

SERVES 4

Preheat the oven to 200°C (400°F) Gas 6.

Toss the pumpkin in 1 tablespoon of the oil and season, then spread out evenly in a large roasting pan. Roast for 30–35 minutes, turning once, until tender and starting to turn golden in places.

Meanwhile, put the freekeh in a pan and cover with water. Bring to the boil, then turn the heat down, cover and simmer for 15 minutes or until tender. Drain and transfer to a serving bowl.

Heat the remaining oil in a frying pan/skillet over a medium heat and fry the ginger for 3 minutes, until crisp and golden. Remove from the pan with a slotted spoon, drain on paper towels and set aside. Add the onion to the pan and fry for 8 minutes, stirring regularly, until softened. Add the garlic and cook for a further minute.

Stir the onion and garlic into the freekeh with the sultanas/golden raisins, orange zest and juice, allspice and ginger. Add a squeeze of lemon juice and the chopped coriander/cilantro, season well, and stir until combined. Serve, sprinkled with the crispy ginger and whole coriander/cilantro leaves.

Spelt is an ancient grain that is a relative of wheat. It isn't technically gluten-free, so those with coeliac disease should substitute buckwheat in this recipe. However, many with wheat sensitivity are able to eat spelt berries because the gluten is more soluble and easy to digest than that present in wheat. Pears and prosciutto are great vehicles for excellent balsamic vinegars. The best ones come from Modena in Italy.

spelt and spinach salad with pear and prosciutto

200 g/1 cup spelt berries
a handful of fresh thyme leaves
100 g/4 cups baby spinach, chopped
2 pears, sliced
12 slices prosciutto or Parma ham
sea salt and freshly ground black
    pepper, to taste

Dressing
3½ tablespoons balsamic vinegar
6 tablespoons olive oil

SERVES 4

Soak the spelt berries in water overnight. Drain and put in a saucepan or pot. Pour in 460 ml/2 cups of water (making sure it's enough to cover the spelt berries). Bring to the boil over a high heat then reduce the temperature, cover and simmer for 45 minutes. Remove the lid and drain if there is any excess water. Put in a separate bowl and leave to cool.

While the spelt berries are cooling, make the dressing by whisking 2 tablespoons of the balsamic vinegar together with the olive oil.

Dress the spelt berries with the balsamic vinaigrette and sprinkle in the fresh thyme leaves. Mix in the spinach. Season with salt and pepper.

To build the salad, scatter the spelt, spinach and thyme mixture on a serving plate. Layer the sliced pears and prosciutto on top.

Drizzle the extra 1½ tablespoons of balsamic vinegar over the pears and prosciutto and serve immediately.

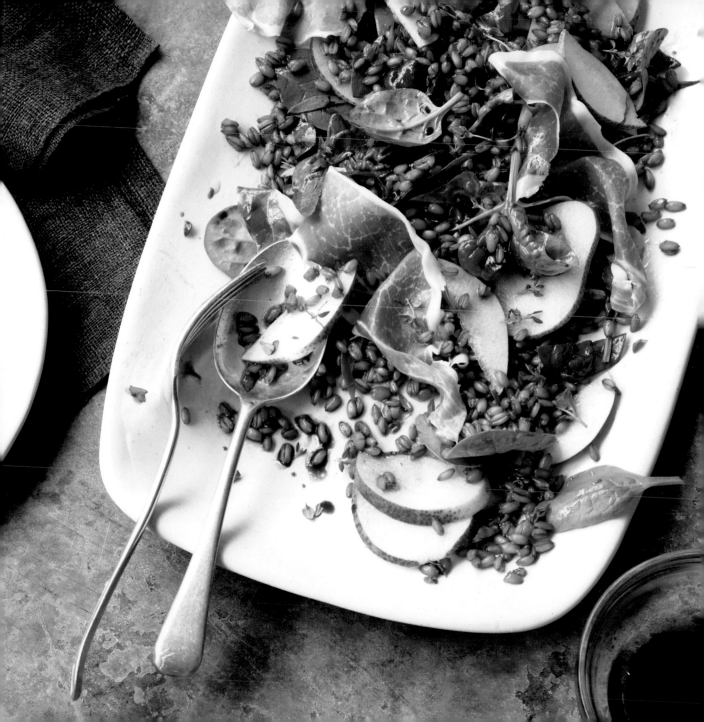

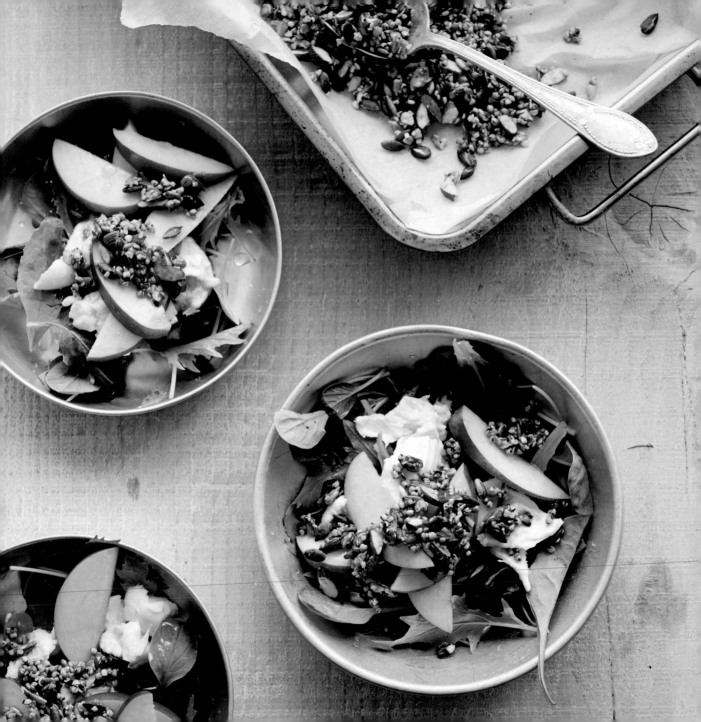

The savoury granola adds a nutritious, nutty crunch to this salad. It's worth making double the quantity to eat as a snack or perhaps sprinkle over yogurt for breakfast. If serving atop sweet dishes, simply omit the tamari sauce and store any leftover granola in an airtight container.

mixed leaves with savoury granola

150 g/5 oz. mixed salad leaves

2 nectarines, halved, stoned/pitted
   and sliced

125 g/4¼ oz. mozzarella, drained and
   torn into pieces

3 tablespoons extra virgin olive oil

freshly squeezed juice of ½ lemon

sea salt and freshly ground black
   pepper, to taste

Savoury granola

1 tablespoon buckwheat groats

1 tablespoon shelled hemp seeds

2 tablespoons sunflower seeds

2 tablespoons pumpkin seeds

a large handful of blanched almonds

1½ teaspoons tamari or light soy
   sauce

1½ teaspoons clear honey

SERVES 4

To make the savoury granola, toast the buckwheat and hemp seeds in a large, dry frying pan/skillet over a medium heat for 2–3 minutes, tossing the pan regularly, until they start to smell toasted. Transfer to a bowl and add the sunflower and pumpkin seeds to the pan. Toast the seeds, again tossing the pan regularly, for 4–5 minutes, until starting to turn golden, then add to the bowl. Finally, add the almonds to the pan and toast for 5 minutes, turning occasionally, until starting to colour. Roughly chop the nuts and add to the bowl with the seeds.

Add the tamari and honey to the nuts and seeds and stir until combined, then leave to cool.

Meanwhile, put the salad leaves in a large serving dish or individual bowls and add the nectarines and mozzarella. Drizzle the olive oil and lemon juice over and season with salt and pepper. Gently toss to combine the ingredients, then sprinkle the granola over before serving.

2 raw beetroot/beets, skin on
a large handful of green beans
100 g/1 cup quinoa
250 ml/1 cup vegetable stock
a handful of toasted pistachios
200 g/1 1/2 cups canned chickpeas
2 oranges, peeled and sliced into
    thin rounds
sea salt and freshly ground black
    pepper, to taste

Shallot crisps
1 shallot, finely sliced
3 tablespoons seasoned chickpea/
    gram flour
vegetable oil for frying

Spicy ginger dressing
grated zest and freshly squeezed juice
    of 1/2 an orange
freshly squeezed juice of 1/2 a lemon
1 garlic clove, crushed
2-cm/3/4-inch piece of fresh ginger,
    finely chopped or grated
1/2–1 fresh red chilli/chile, finely diced
a handful of finely chopped fresh mint

SERVES 2–4

This exotic salad uses quinoa, an excellent, gluten-free alternative to staples such as couscous. For an extra crunchy texture, sprinkle the salad with shallot crisps – they make a great topping for soups, too.

beetroot, quinoa and green bean salad with spicy ginger dressing and shallot crisps

Preheat the oven to 200°C (400°F) Gas 6.

Wrap the beetroot/beets in foil and roast in the preheated oven for 30 minutes, until softened. Allow to cool and cut into bite-size pieces.

Bring a saucepan of water to the boil and cook the green beans for about 4 minutes until they are just cooked but still have a little bite. Plunge them into a bowl of cold water to stop the cooking process and set aside.

Put the quinoa and vegetable stock in a saucepan. Bring to the boil, then simmer for about 15 minutes until the grains are cooked and the stock has been absorbed. Remove from the heat, cover the pan and let the quinoa steam for 5 minutes, then fluff up with a fork.

To make the shallot crisps, toss the sliced shallot in the flour to coat. Pour 1 cm/3/8 inch of oil into a deep pan or wok and set over medium-high heat. Drop the coated shallot slices into the hot oil and fry for 30 seconds until they are crisp and golden. Drain on paper towels and sprinkle with salt.

To make the dressing, put all of the ingredients in a bowl and whisk until well incorporated. Season with salt and pepper.

To assemble the salad, put all the ingredients into a large bowl. Toss with the dressing, then serve on plates with a sprinkling of shallot crisps.

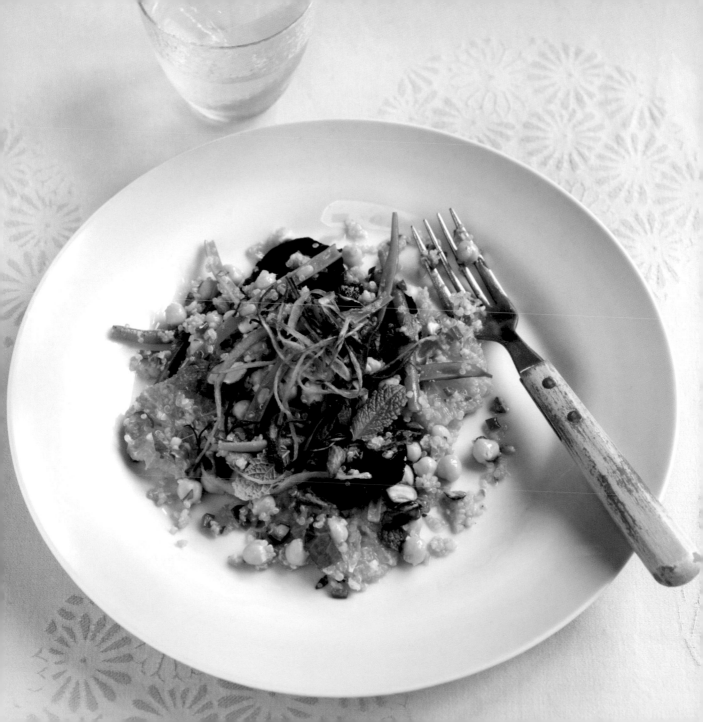

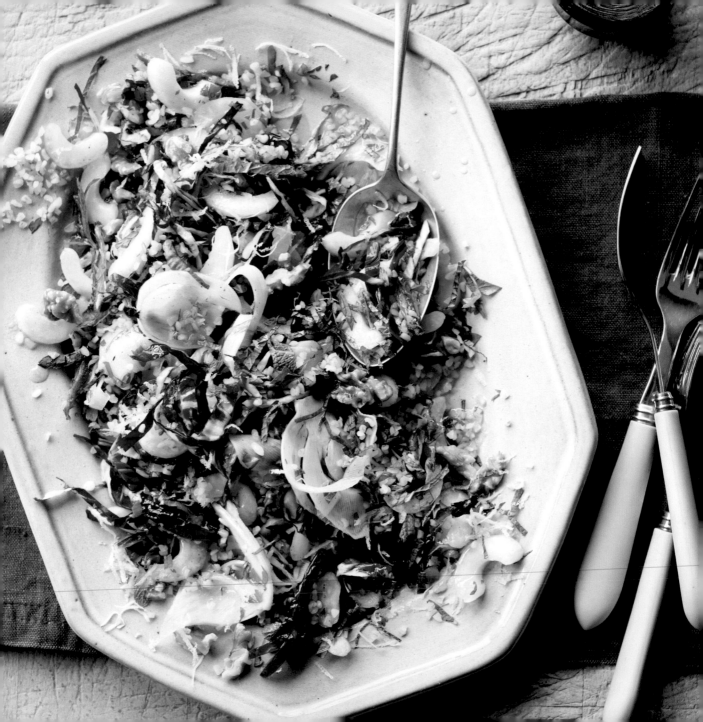

This is a salad of contrasts. Sweet and bitter, soft and crunchy, and a rainbow of colours. Hearty enough as lunch on its own and perfect as an accompaniment to roast chicken or turkey. Bulgur is low in calories but high in fibre/fiber, so you'll still feel full.

crunchy bulgur salad

250 g/1½ cups coarse bulgur

200 g/7 oz. fennel bulb, trimmed and finely diced

freshly squeezed juice and grated zest of ½ lemon

200 g/1½ cups celery, thinly sliced on a diagonal

100 g/¾ cup dried pitted dates, roughly chopped

½ small radicchio, cored and leaves finely shredded

75 g/¾ cup walnuts, roughly chopped

20 g/scant ½ cup roughly chopped fresh flat-leaf parsley

20 g/scant ½ cup roughly chopped fresh mint

sea salt and freshly ground black pepper, to taste

Dressing

1 garlic clove

1 teaspoon sea salt

2 teaspoons pomegranate molasses

50 ml/3 tablespoons olive oil

1 teaspoon ground cinnamon

SERVES 6

Begin by making the dressing. Crush the garlic to a paste with the salt in a pestle and mortar. Transfer to a small mixing bowl and whisk with the remaining ingredients. Cover and set aside.

Put the bulgur in a separate large mixing bowl. Add just enough boiling water to wet the grains but not to submerge them. Cover with clingfilm/plastic wrap and set aside for 15–20 minutes, until just tender but still with a bit of bite. Drain off any excess moisture using a fine mesh sieve/strainer, if necessary.

Put the diced fennel in another large mixing bowl and dress immediately with the lemon juice and zest to prevent any discolouration. Add the remaining ingredients and the soaked bulgur.

Pour over the prepared dressing and season with extra salt and pepper, to taste. Serve on a large plate with salad spoons.

A mix of seasonal mushrooms will give this salad a rich, earthy taste while the dried chilli/hot red pepper flakes adds a welcome touch of warming spice on a cold day.

winter salad of barley, mushrooms and walnuts

200 g/1 cup hulled barley

400 ml/1¾ cups vegetable stock

a handful of shelled walnut halves

1 tablespoon walnut oil

320 g/about 5 cups sliced mixed
    seasonal mushrooms

2 garlic cloves, crushed

¼ teaspoon dried rosemary

¼ teaspoon dried chilli/hot red
    pepper flakes

a handful of peppery salad leaves

sea salt and freshly ground black
    pepper, to taste

Vinaigrette dressing

4 spring onions/scallions, finely
    chopped

2 tablespoons walnut oil

2 teaspoons balsamic vinegar

a squeeze of lemon juice

a handful of finely chopped fresh
    flat-leaf parsley

SERVES 2–4

Put the barley and stock in a saucepan set over a medium heat. Bring to the boil and simmer for 20–30 minutes until the barley is tender but retains its bite.

Meanwhile, toast the walnuts in a dry frying pan/skillet set over a medium heat for 2–3 minutes until golden.

Heat the walnut oil in a separate frying pan/skillet and add the mushrooms and garlic. Fry until golden, then season with salt and pepper. Stir in the rosemary and dried chilli/hot red pepper flakes. Pour the mixture into a bowl and return the pan back to a low heat to make the dressing.

To make the dressing, put the spring onions/scallions, walnut oil, balsamic vinegar and lemon juice in the pan and stir until well combined. Cook until the mixture bubbles. Remove from the heat, season with salt and pepper and stir in the parsley.

To assemble the salad, put the salad leaves in a large bowl with the mushrooms and barley and stir in the dressing. Toss to combine, spoon into serving bowls and serve immediately.

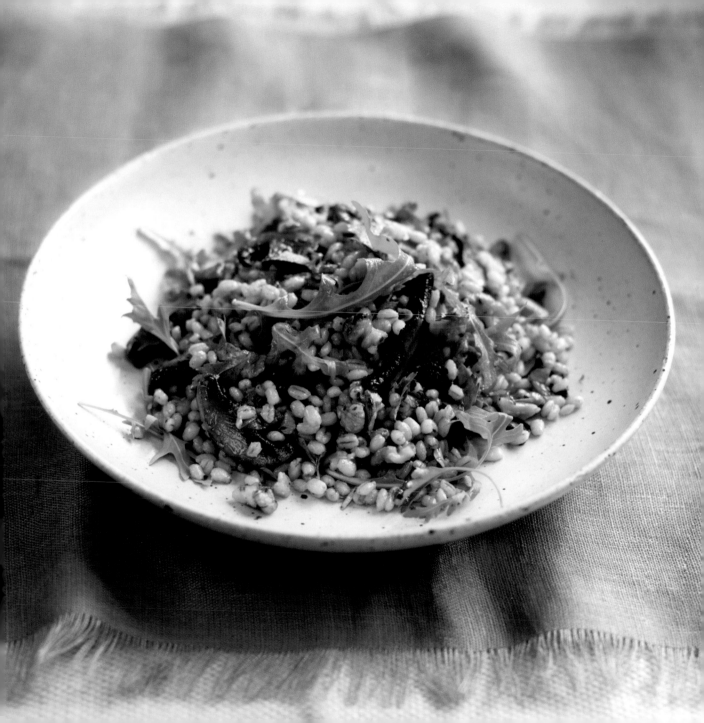

Quinoa makes a nutritious alternative to the more usual bulgur wheat in a tabbouleh. The secret to a successful tabbouleh is to get the right balance of grain to fresh produce; too much of the former makes for a slightly dull salad, so be generous with the herbs and vegetables.

red quinoa tabbouleh

125 g/4¼ oz. red quinoa

6 vine-ripened tomatoes, quartered,
   seeded and chopped

2 small Lebanese cucumbers,
   quartered lengthways and diced

4 spring onions/scallions, finely
   chopped

1 courgette/zucchini, coarsely
   grated

6 tablespoons freshly chopped mint

6 tablespoons freshly chopped flat-
   leaf parsley

Dressing

3 tablespoons extra virgin olive oil

4 tablespoons freshly squeezed
   lemon juice

a pinch of cumin seeds

sea salt and freshly ground black
   pepper, to taste

SERVES 4

Put the quinoa in a pan and cover with water. Bring to the boil, then
turn the heat down and simmer, covered, for 10–15 minutes until
tender. Drain using a fine mesh sieve/strainer, transfer the quinoa
to a serving bowl and leave to cool slightly.

Meanwhile, mix together all the ingredients for the dressing and
season to taste.

Add the tomatoes, cucumbers, spring onions/scallions, courgette/
zucchini and herbs to the quinoa. Pour the dressing over and toss
to combine. Check the seasoning and serve at room temperature.

LARGER PLATES

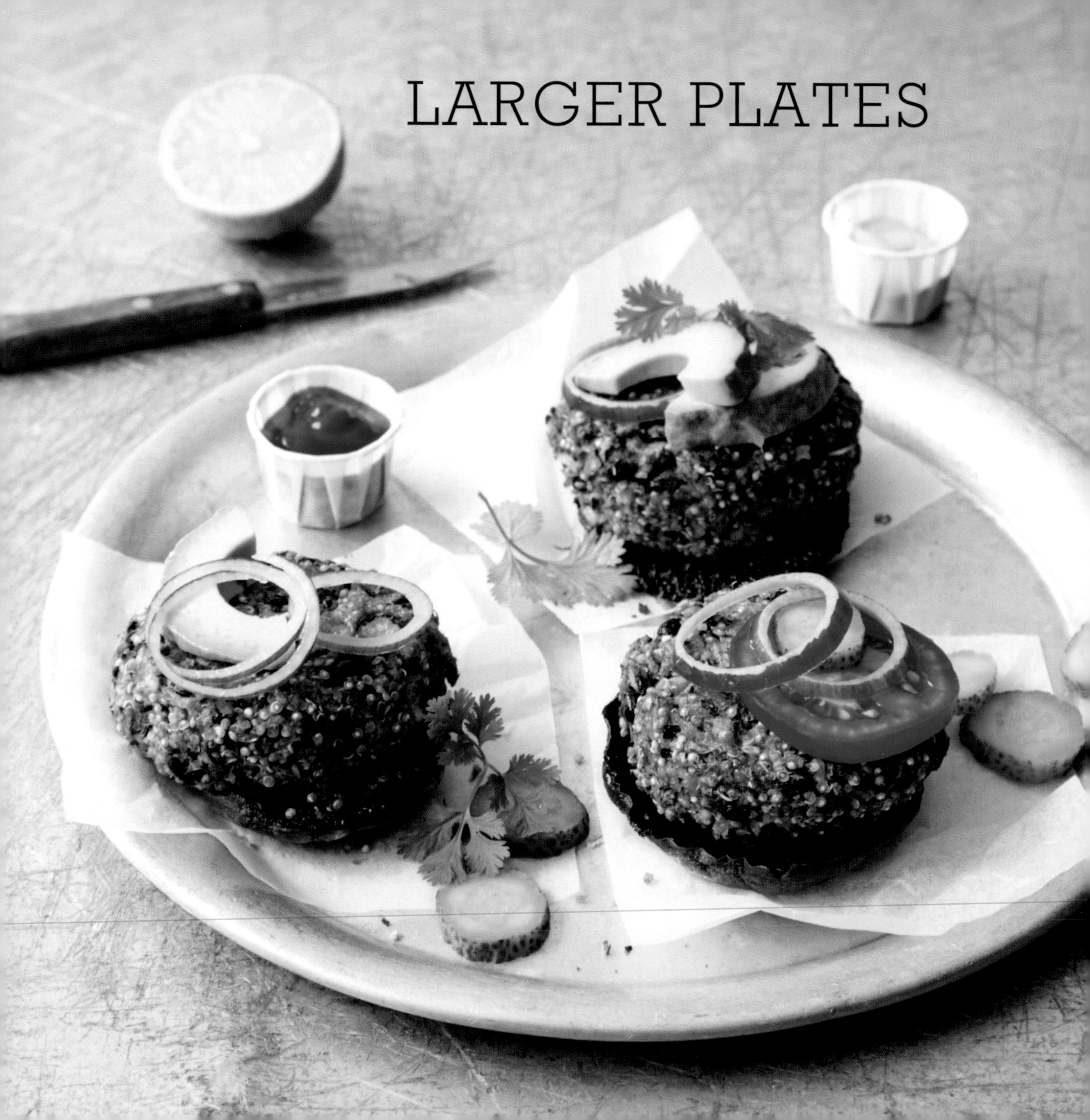

Quinoa is moist and mixes with sweet potato and black beans to give a meaty consistency. Packed full of protein, iron and potassium, this recipe also gives you a boost of anti-oxidants for energy from the black beans.

3 tablespoons olive oil

1 onion, finely chopped

2 garlic cloves, crushed

75 g/½ cup canned black beans

120 g/1 cup cooked quinoa (see Note, page 16)

100 g/½ cup cooked sweet potato flesh

1 carrot, grated

½ teaspoon ground cumin

½ teaspoon ground coriander

2 tablespoons freshly chopped parsley

15 g/⅛ cup gluten-free breadcrumbs

5 portobello mushrooms

a pinch each of sea salt and freshly ground black pepper, to taste

To serve

1 avocado, sliced

1 large tomato, sliced

1 gherkin/pickle, chopped

½ red onion, sliced

a handful of fresh coriander/cilantro

1–2 tablespoons squeezed lime juice

a baking sheet lined with baking parchment

MAKES 5

quinoa burgers with portobello mushrooms

Preheat the oven to 180°C (350°F) Gas 4.

Heat 1 tablespoon of the olive oil in a saucepan set over a medium heat. Add the onion and fry for about 3 minutes, until softened. Add the garlic and cook for another minute. Then add the beans, stir and cook for a few minutes longer. Remove from the heat and transfer the mixture to a large mixing bowl.

Lightly mash the beans with a fork until they're semi-crushed. Add the rest of the ingredients (except the mushrooms and remaining olive oil) to the bowl and mix well. If the mixture is too moist, add extra breadcrumbs. If too dry, add some more mashed beans.

Form five patties with your hands and place on the prepared baking sheet. Bake in the preheated oven for 20–25 minutes, checking after about 15 minutes and turning once to ensure even browning. Once cooked, remove from the main oven and keep warm in a cool oven or on a hot plate.

Increase the temperature of the oven to 200°C (400°F) Gas 6.

For the mushroom base, clean the mushrooms with a damp cloth. Remove the stems and drizzle with the remaining 2 tablespoons olive oil. Season with salt and pepper and roast for 20 minutes.

When ready to serve, place each burger on top of a roasted mushroom and garnish with your choice of traditional burger toppings.

400 g/14 oz. vine-ripened cherry
tomatoes
1 tablespoon extra virgin olive oil
150 g/5 oz. kamut
200 g/7 oz. spring greens/collards or
kale, tough outer leaves and stems
discarded, leaves finely shredded
2 large handfuls of freshly chopped
coriander/cilantro leaves

Chermoula dressing
1 small preserved lemon and
2 tablespoons juice from the jar
4 tablespoons extra virgin olive oil
2 garlic cloves, crushed
1 teaspoon each ground cumin,
ground ginger and ground
coriander
½ teaspoon dried chilli/hot red
pepper flakes
sea salt and freshly ground
black pepper, to taste

SERVES 4

Kamut, or khorasan wheat, is an ancient type of Middle Eastern wheat which is experiencing a resurgence in popularity, but you can use barley or brown rice instead.

kamut with chermoula dressing

Preheat the oven to 200°C (400°F) Gas 6.

Toss the tomatoes in the oil and spread out in a large roasting pan. Roast for 15–20 minutes, until starting to collapse.

Meanwhile, put the kamut in a pan and cover with plenty of water. Bring to the boil, then turn the heat down, part-cover and simmer for 10–12 minutes, until tender. Drain and transfer to a serving bowl with the spring greens/collards and coriander/cilantro.

For the dressing, scoop out and discard the flesh from the preserved lemon. Finely chop the skin and combine it with the rest of the ingredients in a bowl. Season with salt and pepper. Spoon half of the dressing over the salad and toss to combine. Pile the tomatoes on top, then spoon over the rest of the dressing and serve.

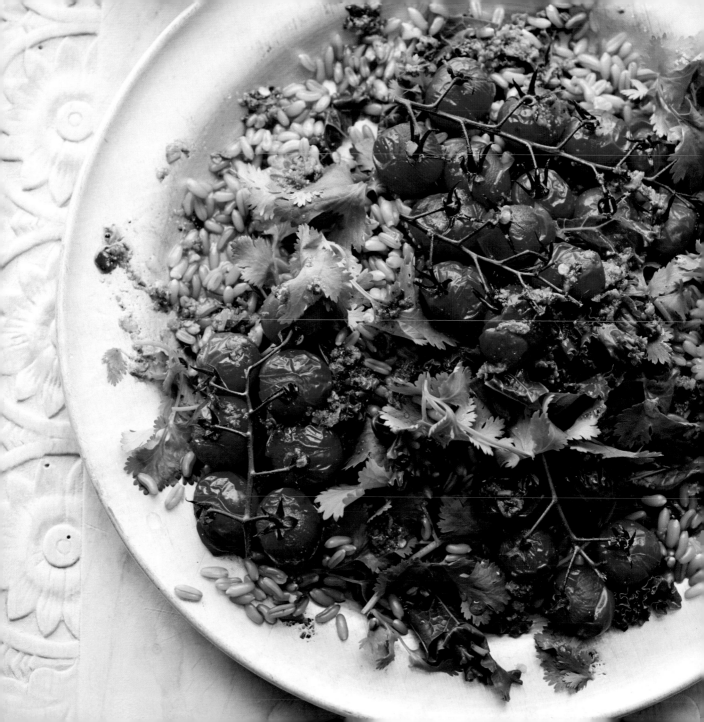

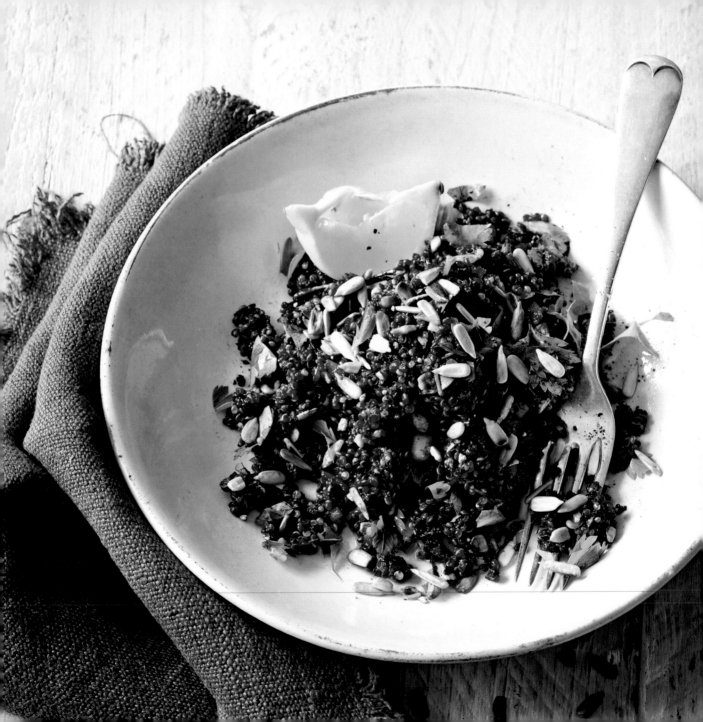

This simple, bright-pink dish is ideal as a light summer supper. Once made, it can sit in the fridge for two days – the flavours will develop and it will become even more delicious over time.

beetroot and quinoa bowl

2 medium beetroot/beets, weighing around 400 g/14 oz.

¼ teaspoon salt

170 g/1 cup quinoa

480 ml/2 cups water

70 g/½ cup sunflower seeds, shelled, rinsed under cold running water and drained

1 tablespoon umeboshi vinegar

1 small onion, finely chopped

4 tablespoons olive oil

freshly squeezed lemon juice or apple cider vinegar, to taste

4 tablespoons freshly chopped flat-leaf parsley

sea salt and freshly ground black pepper, to taste

a pickle press (optional)

a 1-litre/quart preserving jar

SERVES 4

Wash, peel and finely grate the beetroot/beets. Put in a bowl, add the salt and squeeze really well with your hands until the flesh starts 'sweating'. Cover with a small plate that fits into the bowl, top with a weight, and allow to rest for 24 hours. If you have a small pickle press, use this instead. If there isn't enough juice to cover the beetroot/beets, add just enough salted water to cover. Drain off most of the pickle juice before using.

Put the quinoa in a sieve/strainer and rinse well under running water. Drain. Put the drained quinoa into the preserving jar covered with 480 ml/2 cups water. Loosely cover the jar with a lid or with muslin/cheesecloth with a rubber band tied around it. Soak for 24 hours at room temperature.

Put both the quinoa and the soaking water in a saucepan, bring to a boil, add a few pinches of salt, lower the heat to its minimum setting, half-cover the saucepan and cook for about 15 minutes, until the quinoa absorbs all the water. Remove from the heat and allow to cool.

Put the sunflower seeds in a frying pan/skillet over a medium heat and dry-roast, stirring vigorously until the seeds start sizzling and turn golden brown. Pour into a clean bowl and, while still hot, pour over the umeboshi vinegar and stir until absorbed. If you don't have umeboshi vinegar, dissolve ¼ teaspoon of salt in ½ tablespoon hot water and pour over the seeds. Stir until absorbed.

In a large glass mixing bowl, gently mix all the ingredients except for the parsley and season with the olive oil, some lemon juice or cider vinegar, salt and pepper. Garnish with the chopped parsley. Refrigerate before serving.

165 g/5½ oz. green lentils, rinsed

4 tablespoons amaranth

6 spring onions/scallions, sliced

6 vine-ripened tomatoes, roughly
    chopped

1 yellow courgette/zucchini, coarsely
    grated

2 handfuls of freshly chopped mint
    leaves, plus a few whole leaves
    to decorate

1 tablespoon Za'atar (see below)

Za'atar

3 tablespoons thyme leaves

2 teaspoons sumac

½ teaspoon sea salt

1 tablespoon sesame seeds, toasted

Dressing

2 tablespoons pomegranate molasses

3 tablespoons extra virgin olive oil

finely grated zest and freshly
    squeezed juice of 1 lemon

sea salt and freshly ground black
    pepper, to taste

SERVES 4

Popular in South America, amaranth is gluten-free as well as being a good source of valuable minerals. This tiny grain (or, more accurately, seed) packs a powerful nutritional punch for its diminutive size with even more protein than oats.

amaranth and green lentil salad with za'atar

Put the lentils in a large pan and cover with plenty of cold water. Bring to the boil, then turn the heat down and simmer, part-covered, for 20 minutes or until tender. Drain and transfer the lentils to a serving bowl.

Meanwhile, toast the amaranth in a dry pan for 2 minutes, shaking the pan regularly, until the grains start to pop and turn golden. Pour enough water over to cover and bring to the boil, then turn the heat down and simmer for 6 minutes or until tender. Drain and add to the bowl with the lentils.

To make the za'atar, preheat the oven to 160°C (325°F) Gas 3. Put the thyme on a small baking sheet in the oven for 5 minutes, or until dried. Crumble the thyme leaves into a bowl and mix in the sumac, salt and sesame seeds. Let cool and transfer to an airtight container if not using immediately.

Mix together all the dressing ingredients and season to taste.

Add the spring onions/scallions, tomatoes, courgette/zucchini and mint to the serving bowl, and pour enough of the dressing over to coat. Toss until combined and serve, sprinkled with the za'atar and a few whole mint leaves.

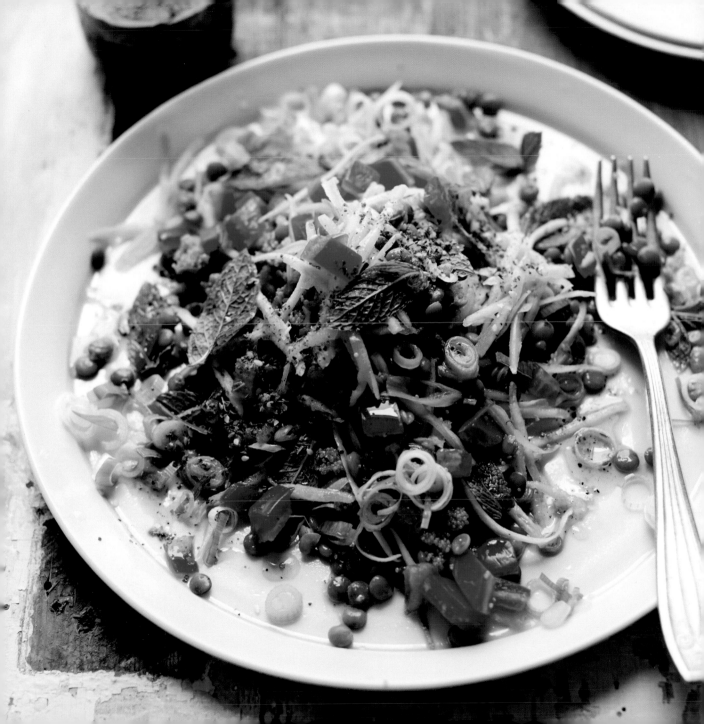

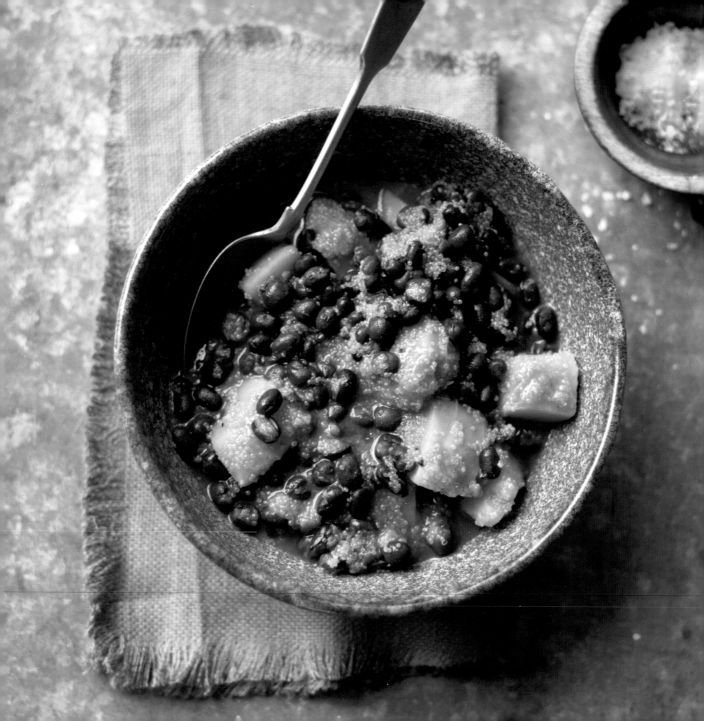

You will feel goodness in your body while eating this stew! It's made with only a handful of ingredients, but the consistency is rich and creamy and the taste slightly sweet. After travelling, not eating well or a stressful day, this stew will take all your worries away!

adzuki bean stew with amaranth

200 g/1 cup dried adzuki beans

180 g/1½ cups peeled, seeded and cubed Hokkaido or kabocha pumpkin

70 g/⅓ cup amaranth

2 tablespoons gluten-free soy sauce or tamari sauce

½ tablespoon umeboshi vinegar

½ teaspoon ground turmeric

½ teaspoon sea salt

SERVES 2–3

Cover the adzuki beans with 1 litre/4 cups of cold water in a saucepan and soak them overnight (this is not necessary but will speed up the cooking). The next day, bring them to a boil in the soaking water, then add the pumpkin and cook, half-covered, over a low heat for about 30 minutes, until the beans are half-done.

Add the amaranth and cook for another 20–30 minutes, until both the beans and amaranth are soft. Season with the remaining ingredients and adjust the thickness by adding hot water, if necessary.

This stew doesn't have any oil and provides the body with a lot of well-balanced nutrients. It is a great winter dish when you feel exhausted and need comfort food that is easy to digest.

Like rice, there are many forms of barley. Hulled barley has most of its outer layer intact, so it is considered a wholegrain. Pearl barley has had its outer layer completely removed so it does not earn its place as a coveted 'supergrain' and does not have the same health benefits. The bran layer contains the fibre/fiber, vitamins and protein. Barley is chewy and mild tasting so it is very versatile. It's great in soups, salads and pilafs. However, it is not gluten-free, so substitute with brown basmati rice for this dish when required.

saffron shrimp with barley pilaf

1 onion, chopped

2 tablespoons plus 1 teaspoon vegetable oil

1 garlic clove, crushed

200 g/1 cup hulled barley

480 ml/2 cups vegetable stock

1 bay leaf

1 teaspoon paprika

1 teaspoon turmeric

1 teaspoon ground cinnamon

1 teaspoon ground cardamom

a pinch of saffron threads

12 medium uncooked prawns/shrimp, peeled and deveined

a handful of fresh flat-leaf parsley, to garnish

SERVES 2

In a medium saucepan or pot, fry the onion in 2 tablespoons of the oil for 4–5 minutes over a high heat. Reduce the heat, then add the garlic and barley, toasting for 3 minutes. Then add 240 ml/1 cup of water, the stock and bay leaf. Bring to the boil, then cover and simmer for about 50 minutes. The grains will be softened and chewy when fully cooked.

In a separate non-stick frying pan/skillet, heat the remaining teaspoon of oil over a medium heat and add the paprika, turmeric, cinnamon, cardamom and saffron. Add the prawns/shrimp and fry for 3 minutes on each side, or until they are completely opaque.

Remove the bay leaf from the barley and scoop a generous amount and 6 prawns/shrimp onto each plate or serving dish. Garnish with fresh flat-leaf parsley and serve.

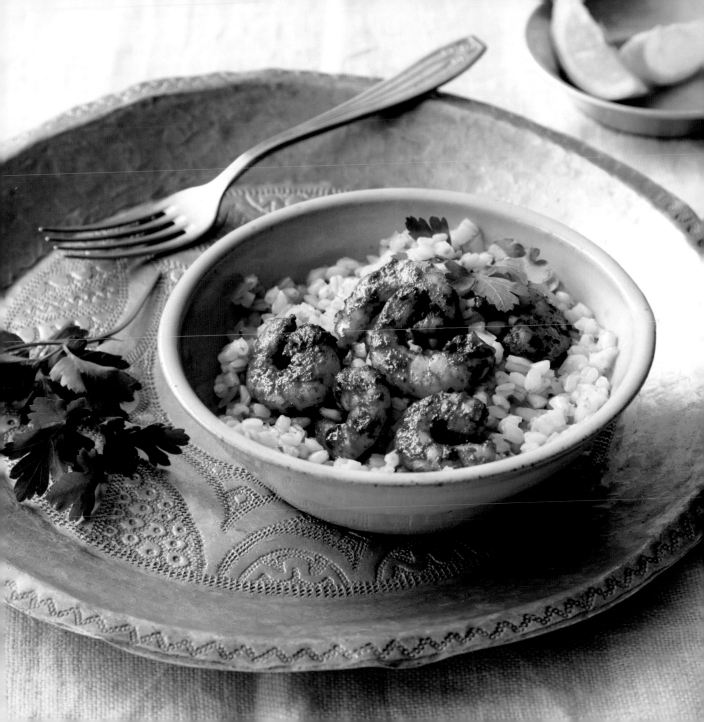

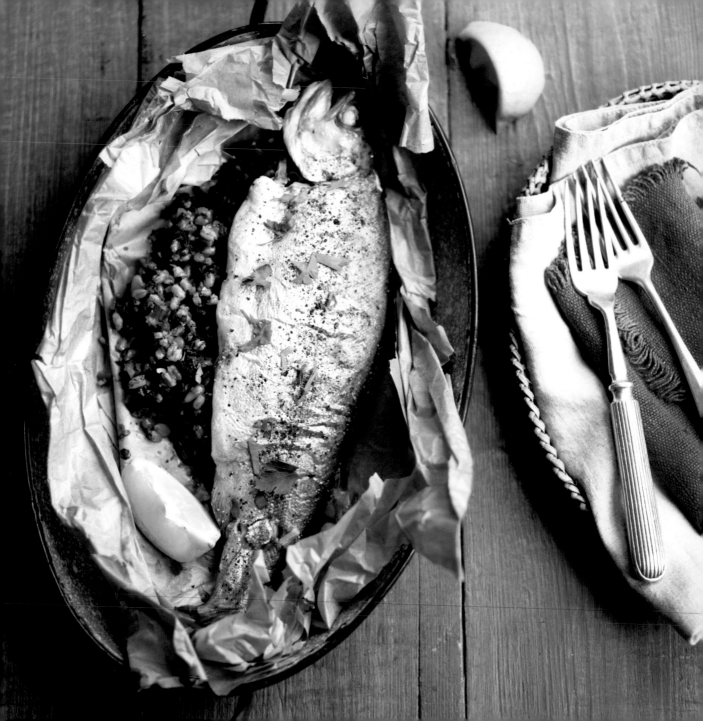

Farro is an ancient grain with a delicious slightly nutty flavour and chewy consistency. It is high in protein and lower in gluten than wheat, so some people with an intolerance to wheat find they tolerate farro. Do not confuse it with spelt, which has a much harder shell and takes far longer to cook. Camargue red rice or short-grain rice could also be used.

trout stuffed with farro, dates and pine nuts

150 g/1 heaped cup farro

1 teaspoon red wine vinegar

3 tablespoons extra virgin olive oil

1 onion, finely chopped

1 garlic clove, crushed

1 handful fresly chopped coriander/ cilantro

1 handful freshly chopped flat-leaf parsley

30 g/¼ cup pine nuts, lightly roasted until golden

4 Medjool dates, pitted/stoned and chopped

2 lemons, 1 zested and halved, the other cut into wedges

2 trout, cleaned, gutted and scaled

sea salt and freshly ground black pepper, to taste

SERVES 4–6

Rinse the farro thoroughly until the water runs clear. Add to a pot of cold water with a pinch of salt. Bring to the boil, then reduce heat and simmer for 20–25 minutes, until al dente. Farro has a natural chewiness to it and you want to keep that texture, so taste it a few times to get the consistency just right. Drain off the water and immediately, while still hot, stir in the red wine vinegar and 2 tablespoons of the olive oil. Season to taste.

Sweat the onion in a frying pan/skillet with the remaining tablespoon of oil over a medium heat until softened. Add in the garlic and cook for a further 1–2 minutes until aromatic. Add the cooked farro and combine together with the coriander/cilantro, most of the parsley, the pine nuts, Medjool dates and lemon zest. Taste and adjust the seasoning if necessary.

Preheat the oven to 200°C (400°F) Gas 6.

Season the trout with salt and pepper, both inside and out. Place on a baking sheet with enough aluminium foil or parchment paper to create a parcel. Stuff the cavity of the fish with the farro, squeeze a little juice from the zested lemon halves around the fish and then nestle the lemon beside them. Seal the parcel tightly and bake in the centre of the oven for 15 minutes. Open the parcel, exposing the fish, and cook for another 5 minutes until the skin is slightly blistered and golden.

Serve on a platter with the lemon wedges and the remaining parsley.

This colourful, healthy dish is packed full of iron from the quinoa and omega-3 fatty acids from the salmon. Capers add a salty zing to balance out the citrus dressing made with clementine.

cold poached salmon with cucumber quinoa salad

1 lemon, sliced

120 ml/$^1/_2$ cup white wine

500 g/2 salmon fillets

1 tablespoon capers

3 small cucumbers, diced

2 tablespoons finely sliced red onion, soaked in water for 10 minutes

$^1/_2$ yellow (bell) pepper, chopped

15 g/8 tablespoons chopped dill

2 tablespoons chopped chives

280 g/2 cups cooked quinoa (see Note, page 16)

Himalayan salt and freshly ground black pepper, to taste

Dressing

4 tablespoons extra virgin olive oil

2 tablespoons champagne vinegar

freshly squeezed juice of 1 clementine or lemon

SERVES 2

Put 4 slices of lemon, 120 ml/$^1/_2$ cup of water and the white wine in a large frying pan/skillet. Place the salmon fillets on top of the lemon slices, skin side down.

Bring the liquid to a simmer over a medium–high heat. Turn the heat to low, cover and cook for 5 minutes. Then turn off the heat, and let the fish sit over the heat for a further 5 minutes while it continues to cook. This is a good way to prevent it from overcooking.

Transfer the salmon fillets to a plate, reserving the poaching liquid.

Add the capers and some salt and pepper to the poaching liquid and reduce by half over a medium heat to make a sauce. Drizzle the sauce over the salmon; cover and chill in the refrigerator.

In a large mixing bowl, mix together the cucumbers, drained red onion, yellow (bell) pepper, 1 tablespoon each of the dill and chives, and the cooked quinoa.

Make the dressing by whisking all of the ingredients together. Then drizzle over the quinoa salad. Plate the salmon with the quinoa salad and garnish with the reserved dill and chives.

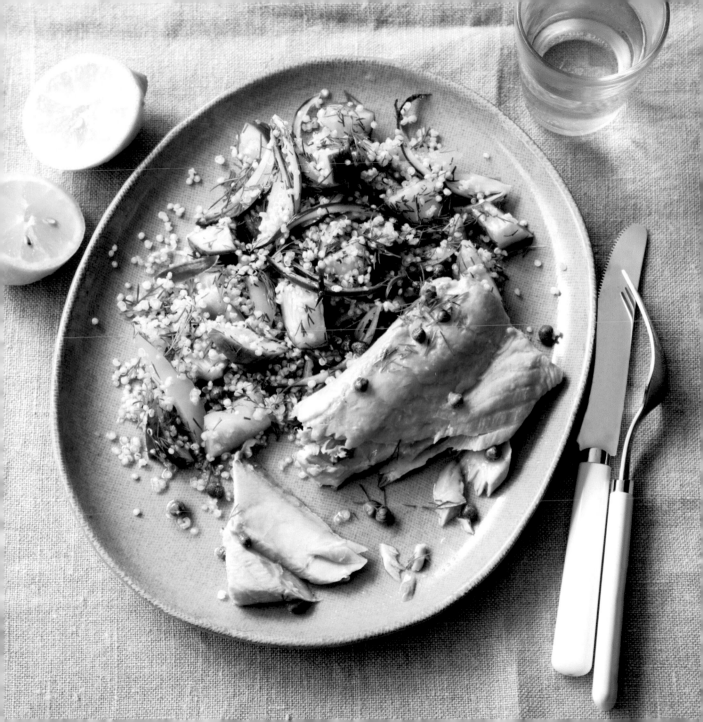

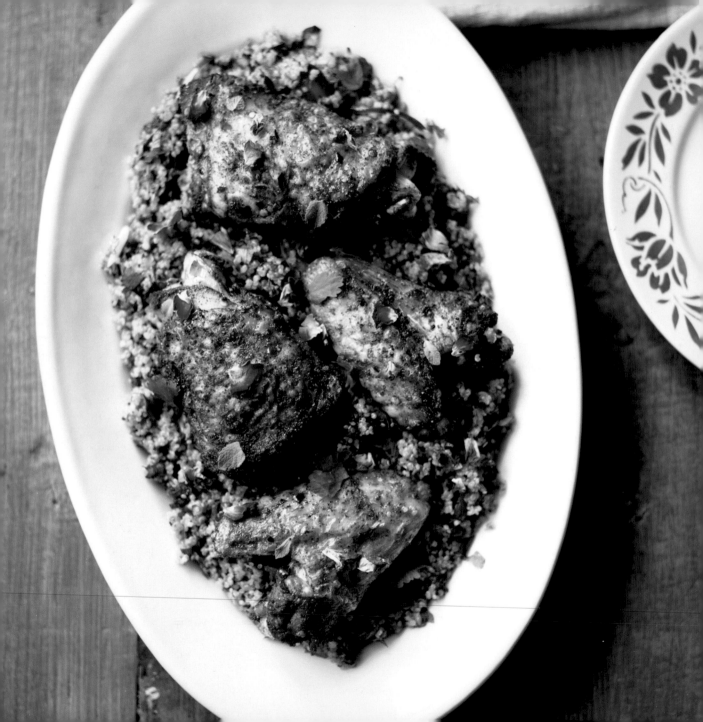

Quinoa is a great base for salads or, like here, spiced up and served with meat or fish. It's a fantastic source of protein, containing all the essential amino acids, and can be used as you would couscous or millet.

spiced chicken with quinoa, lemon zest and rose petals

4 chicken thighs and 4 wings

extra virgin olive oil, to drizzle, plus extra for frying

1 tablespoon *ras el hanout* (spice mix)

1 teaspoon dried chilli/hot red pepper flakes

1 red onion, halved and thinly sliced

1 teaspoon ground cinnamon

1 teaspoon ground cumin

3 garlic cloves, crushed

250 g/1¼ cups quinoa

12 dried apricots, sliced

grated zest of ½ lemon

1 handful each of freshly chopped flat-leaf parsley, mint and coriander/cilantro leaves, plus some whole leaves to serve

1 tablespoon pomegranate molasses or lemon juice

sea salt and freshly ground black pepper, to taste

rose petals (optional)

SERVES 4–6

Preheat the oven to 190°C (375°F) Gas 5.

Place the chicken in a large roasting pan and drizzle over 1 tablespoon of olive oil, just enough to coat them. Season with plenty of sea salt and sprinkle over the *ras el hanout* and chilli/hot red pepper flakes. Use your hands to massage the spices into the chicken. Roast for 25–30 minutes or until cooked through and the skin is crisp and golden. Keep warm.

In a large saucepan, gently sauté the red onion in a little olive oil until soft. Add in the cinnamon, cumin, garlic and 1 teaspoon salt and fry for another couple of minutes until aromatic. Add in the quinoa and just under double its quantity of water, about 500 ml/2 cups. Bring to a boil, then reduce the heat to low and place the lid on top. Cook for about 12 minutes, then remove the lid and continue to cook until all the water has been absorbed and the quinoa is quite dry. Turn off the heat and add in the sliced apricots and lemon zest. Stir in the herbs, pomegranate molasses (or lemon juice), and season to taste with salt and pepper. Gently combine together.

Plate up the quinoa with the chicken on top and remaining herbs and rose petals scattered over, if using.

BAKES

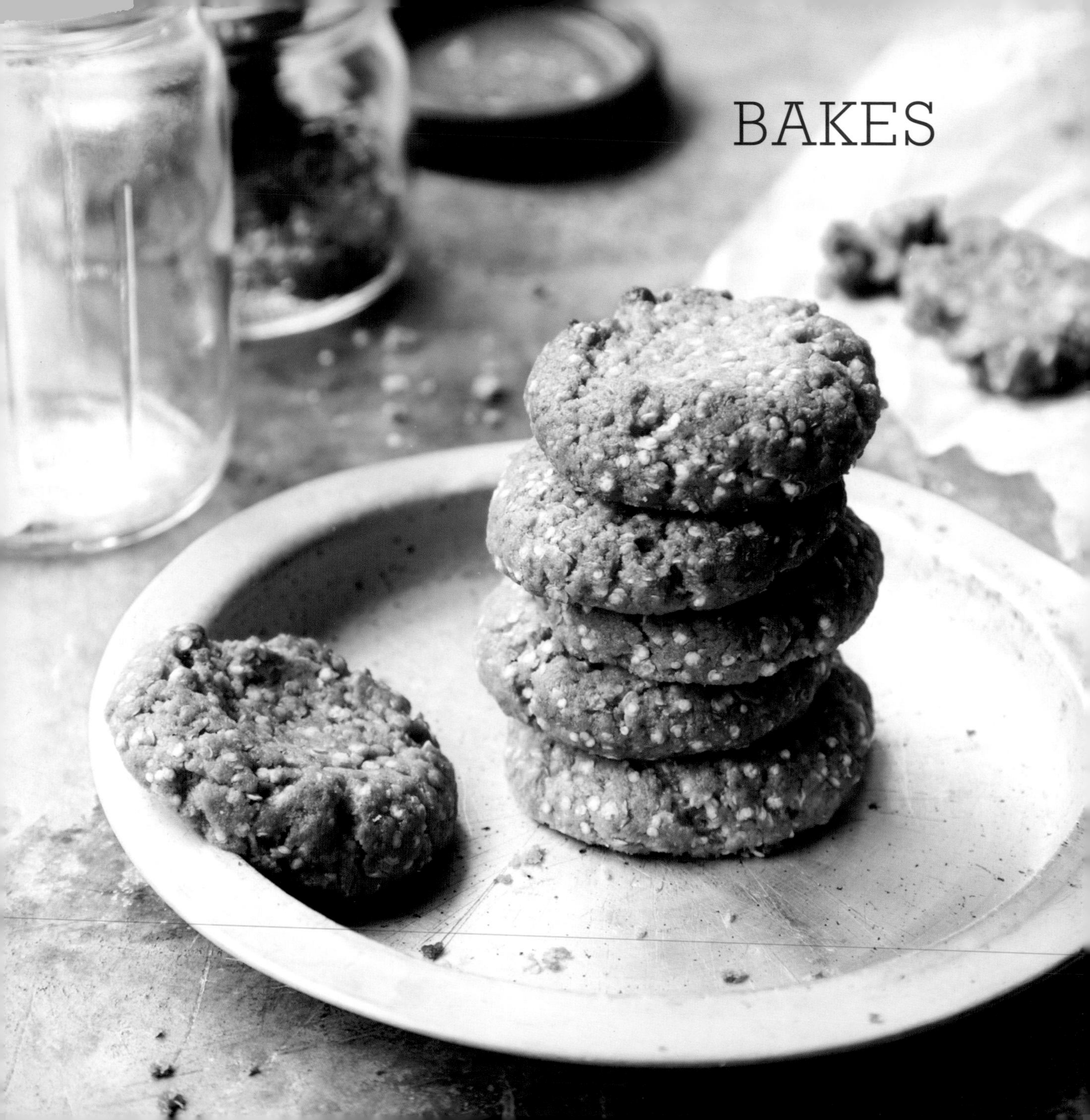

These are good – really good. You will use quinoa in its flake and flour form for a double power grain boost.

peanut butter quinoa cookies

420 g/1¾ cup creamy peanut butter

75 g/¾ cup xylitol or other sugar substitute

140 ml/¾ cup agave syrup

2 eggs (see Note)

1 teaspoon vanilla extract

45 g/½ cup quinoa flakes

2 tablespoons quinoa flour

½ teaspoon bicarbonate of soda/ baking soda

a baking sheet lined with baking parchment

MAKES 24

Preheat the oven to 180°C (350°F) Gas 4.

Mix all ingredients together in a large mixing bowl. Once the ingredients are all combined, bring the mixture together in your hands then roll into 2.5-cm/1-inch balls and place onto the prepared baking sheet. Using your thumb, press down each ball so it is slightly flattened out.

Bake in the preheated oven for about 12 minutes, until the cookies are golden, and serve warm.

Store the cookies in an airtight container for up to 3 days.

Note: If you prefer not to use eggs you could use egg replacer or make a flax-egg mix by combining 2 tablespoons of ground flaxseed with 6 tablespoons of water.

This tart is all about the blueberries – a blueberry compote lines the tart and then a small mountain of tumbling blueberries are heaped on top. It's best served chilled on a summer's day when the fruit is in season.

fresh blueberry tart

225 g/1²⁄₃ cups white spelt flour

¼ teaspoons sea salt

120 g/generous ½ cup coconut palm sugar, plus 1 tablespoon

50 g/3 tablespoons dairy-free butter (e.g. sunflower spread), cut into small chunks

60 g/4 tablespoons vegetable fat/ shortening, cut into small chunks

1 egg, beaten together with 1 teaspoon water

2 tablespoons cornflour/cornstarch

finely grated zest of 1 lemon and 1 tablespoon freshly squeezed juice

900 g/2 lbs. blueberries

small handful of fresh mint leaves

1 teaspoon xylitol, ground to a fine powder

dairy-free yogurt or ice cream, to serve (optional)

a 25-cm/10-inch tart pan, greased

SERVES 10–12

Sift the flour into a large bowl. Add the salt and 1 tablespoon of coconut palm sugar. With your hands high, rub the dairy-free butter and vegetable fat/shortening into the flour until it resembles breadcrumbs.

Slowly add in the egg and water mixture a tablespoon at a time, forking the mixture together as you go. Bring the dough together with your hands to form a smooth ball. If it is still crumbly and not coming together, add a little bit more liquid, being careful not to overdo it. Gently flatten into a round, wrap in clingfilm/plastic wrap and put in the fridge until very cold.

Preheat the oven to 180°C (360°F) Gas 4.

Once the pastry is cold, roll it out and line the prepared tart pan. You can roll it between 2 sheets of clingfilm/plastic wrap to make it easier. Bake the tart blind for about 20 minutes. Remove the blind baking weights and return to the oven for a further 5–10 minutes until the base is dry and biscuity. Remove from the pan and cool on a wire rack.

Stir together the cornflour/cornstarch and lemon juice, making sure there are no lumps, and add to a pan with a little over half of the blueberries, the lemon zest and the remaining coconut palm sugar. Stir over a medium– high heat for 10–15 minutes, squishing the berries as you go, until it is the consistency of a thick, soft jam/jelly. Leave to cool completely, then pour into the cold pastry case and smooth over. Tumble on the remaining blueberries, cover and refrigerate until well chilled.

When ready to serve, scatter over as much mint as you like and dust with ground xylitol. Some dairy-free yogurt or ice cream on the side is delicious.

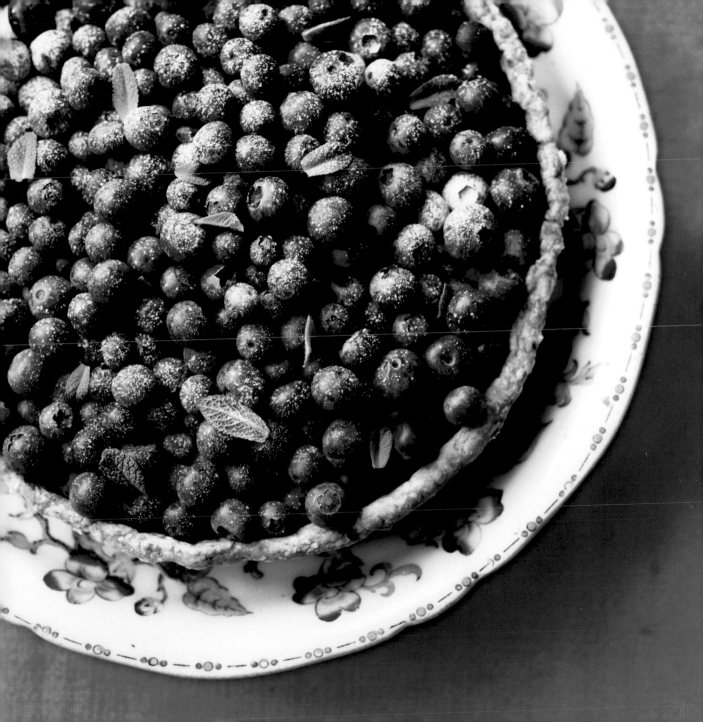

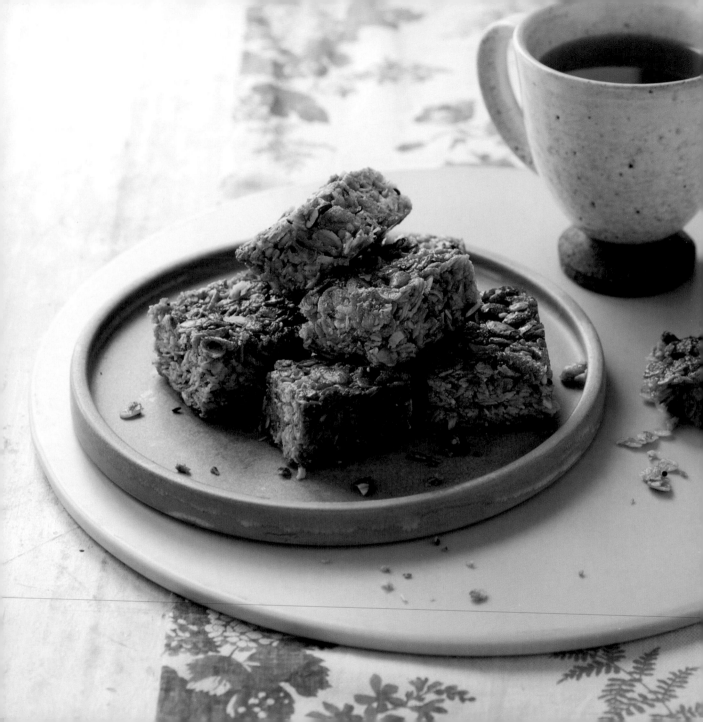

These sticky oat bars are easy to make and packed with oats and seeds, so they make a great accompaniment to a tea or coffee for those who aren't big on breakfast, or are a little short on time in the mornings.

sticky oat breakfast bars

225 g/scant 1 cup unsalted butter
225 g/1 cup plus 2 tablespoons brown sugar
3 tablespoons clear honey
a pinch of salt
325 g/3¼ cups jumbo oats
2 tablespoons mixed seeds (such as sunflower, sesame, hemp, pumpkin or linseeds)
50 g/1 cup cornflakes

a 20 x 30-cm/8 x 12-in baking pan, greased and lined with baking parchment

MAKES 15

Preheat the oven to 180°C (350°F) Gas 4.

Melt the butter, sugar, honey and salt together in a saucepan over gentle heat. Stir in the oats, seeds and cornflakes.

Spoon the mixture into the prepared pan and bake for 20–25 minutes, until golden and firm.

Leave to cool in the pan, then cut into squares.

This wholesome bread tastes wonderfully nutty thanks to the variety of seeds in the mixture. One slice is so hearty and packed with flavour that it will keep you feeling full for a long while!

multigrain seeded bread

20 g/2 tablespoons sesame seeds

20 g/2 tablespoons linseed/flaxseed

20 g/2 tablespoons buckwheat or kasha (roasted buckwheat)

20 g/2 tablespoons sunflower seeds, lightly toasted (optional)

500 g/4 cups wholemeal/whole-wheat flour

10 g/2 teaspoons salt

8 g/2/3 teaspoon fresh yeast or 4 g/1 1/4 teaspoons fast-action dried yeast

80 ml/1/3 cup warm water

a 900-g/8 1/2 x 4 1/2-in. loaf pan, greased with vegetable oil

MAKES 1 LARGE LOAF

Put 300 ml/1 1/4 cups of cold water and the grains and seeds in a large mixing bowl and stir. Cover with an upturned smaller mixing bowl. Set aside in a cool place overnight.

The next day, remove the smaller bowl and put the flour and salt into it.

In another small bowl, weigh out the yeast. Add the warm water and stir until the yeast has dissolved. Mix the yeast solution into the seed mixture, then add the flour mixture and mix by hand until it comes together. Cover with the bowl that had the dry mixture in it. Let stand for 10 minutes.

Knead the dough well for about 20 minutes. Cover the bowl again and let stand for 10 minutes. Repeat the kneading process twice, covering the bowl each time, then knead once more. Cover again and let rise for 1 hour.

Punch down the dough, then turn it out onto a lightly floured work surface. Roll the dough to make a sausage about twice the length of the loaf pan. Shape the sausage into an inverted 'U'. Twist the 2 strands until you reach the end, then place inside the prepared loaf pan. Sprinkle flour over the bread. Cover and let rise until double the size – about 45 minutes.

About 20 minutes before baking, preheat the oven to 240°C (475°F) Gas 9. Place a roasting pan at the bottom of the oven. Fill a cup with water.

Put the risen bread in the preheated oven. Pour the cupful of water onto the hot roasting pan and lower the temperature to 220°C (425°F) Gas 7. Bake for about 30 minutes, or until golden brown. Tip the loaf out of the pan and tap the bottom – it should sound hollow if baked well.

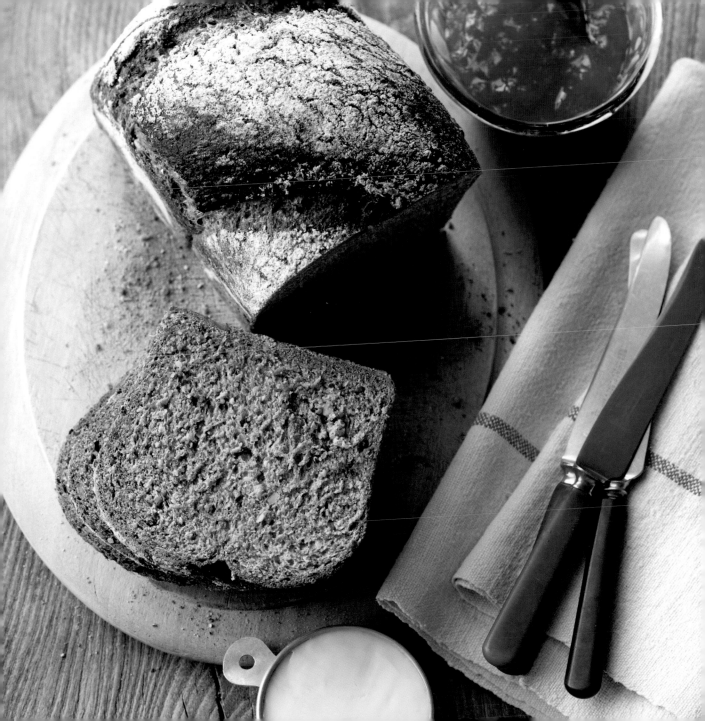

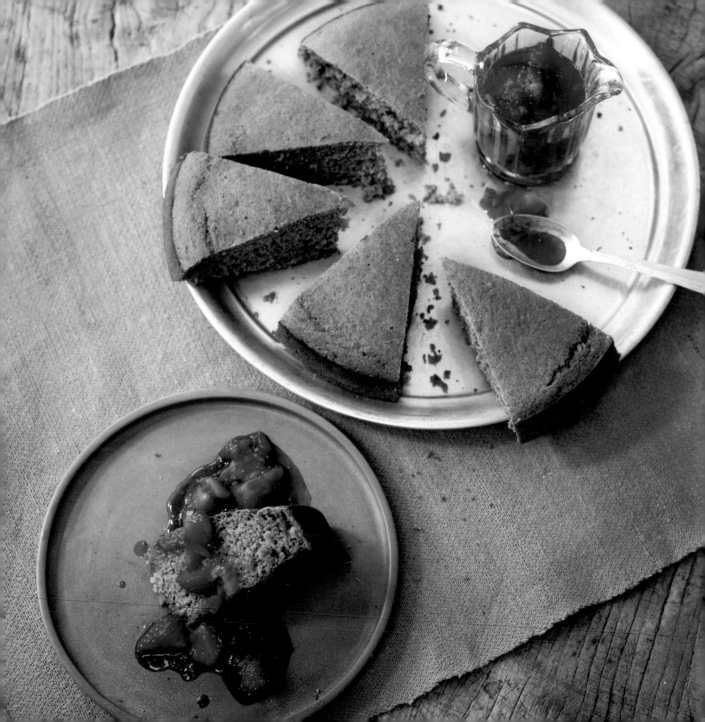

MILLET FLOUR · OAT FLOUR · DAIRY-FREE · VEGAN

This is a lovely light vegan cake to serve at tea parties, topped with fruit coulis or jam/jelly, if fresh berries are out of season. Chestnut flour gives it a subtle nutty aroma, but using cocoa powder, carob powder or coffee powder instead works well, too, and these have the bonus of being great energy boosters.

fluffy cake with strawberry coulis

30 g/¼ cup chestnut flour (or cocoa, carob or coffee powder)
grated zest and juice of 1 lemon
155 ml/²⁄₃ cups soy/soya milk
140 g/1 cup millet (or teff) flour
30 g/¼ cup wholemeal/whole-wheat oat flour
½ teaspoon bicarbonate of soda/baking soda
½ teaspoon baking powder
¼ teaspoon bourbon vanilla powder
⅛ teaspoon sea salt
3 tablespoons sunflower oil
150 g/½ cup rice syrup

Strawberry coulis
320 g/2 cups fresh strawberries
2 tablespoons maple syrup
1 teaspoon lemon juice
a pinch of sea salt

a 24-cm/ 9½-in. springform cake pan, greased and base-lined with baking parchment

If you're using chestnut flour that hasn't been pre-roasted, place it in a dry frying pan/skillet over a medium heat and stir until fragrant. Set aside.

Add the lemon juice to the milk and let sit for 10 minutes. Meanwhile, sift the chestnut, millet and oat flour with the bicarbonate of soda/baking soda and baking powder and then add the vanilla and salt.

Prepare the coulis by mixing all the ingredients and letting them sit for 30 minutes. Mash with a fork to get a juicy coulis with some texture. You can also blend it if you prefer a smooth sauce.

Preheat the oven to 180°C (350°F) Gas 4.

Add the oil and syrup to the milk and lemon mixture and mix well with a spatula. Make sure you don't mix too much, otherwise the cake might turn chewy. Pour the batter into your prepared cake pan and spread evenly.

Bake for 18–20 minutes. Test if done by inserting a cocktail stick/toothpick into the middle of the cake; if it comes out clean, it's done.

Let the cake cool completely, and then cut with a bread knife into 6–8 equal slices. Spoon the coulis over the cake slices just before serving.

index

recipe credits

Jordan Bourke Fresh blueberry tart • Spiced chicken with quinoa, lemon zest and rose petals • Trout stuffed with farro, dates and pine nuts

Chloe Coker and Jane Montgomery Beetroot, quinoa and green bean salad • Winter salad of barley, mushrooms and walnuts

Ross Dobson Fresh shiitake and barley soup

Amy Ruth Finegold Blueberry oat smoothie • Cold poached salmon with cucumber quinoa salad • Fruit and oat muffins • Peanut butter oat shake • Peanut butter quinoa cookies • Quinoa burgers with Portobello mushrooms • Quinoa soup with red beans and kale • Saffron shrimp with barley pilaf • Spelt and spinach salad with pear and prosciutto

Liz Franklin Sticky oat breakfast bars

Nicola Graimes Amaranth and green lentil salad with za'atar • Freekeh, pumpkin and crispy ginger salad • Kamut with chermoula dressing • Mixed leaves with savoury granola • Red quinoa tabbouleh

Dunja Gulin Adzuki bean stew with amaranth • Beetroot and quinoa bowl • Fluffy cake with strawberry coulis

Emmanuel Hadjiandreou Multigrain seeded bread

Carol Hilker Quinoa porridge with maple syrup and brown sugar

Shelagh Ryan Crunchy bulgur salad • Lamb shank broth with barley

Jenna Zoe Power protein granola

picture credits

Key: r - right; l - left; c - centre

Peter Cassidy: 14

Tara Fisher: 4, 38, 48, 52, 53, 57

Richard Jung: 29, 33

Steve Painter: 61

William Reavell: 5r, 44, 62

Matt Russell: 3, 22, 26, 34, 39, 43

Toby Scott: 40

Kate Whitaker : 21, 30

Isobel Wield: 58, 59

Clare Winfield: endpapers, 1, 2, 5c, 6-7, 10, 13, 17, 18, 25, 35, 36, 47, 51, 54, 55

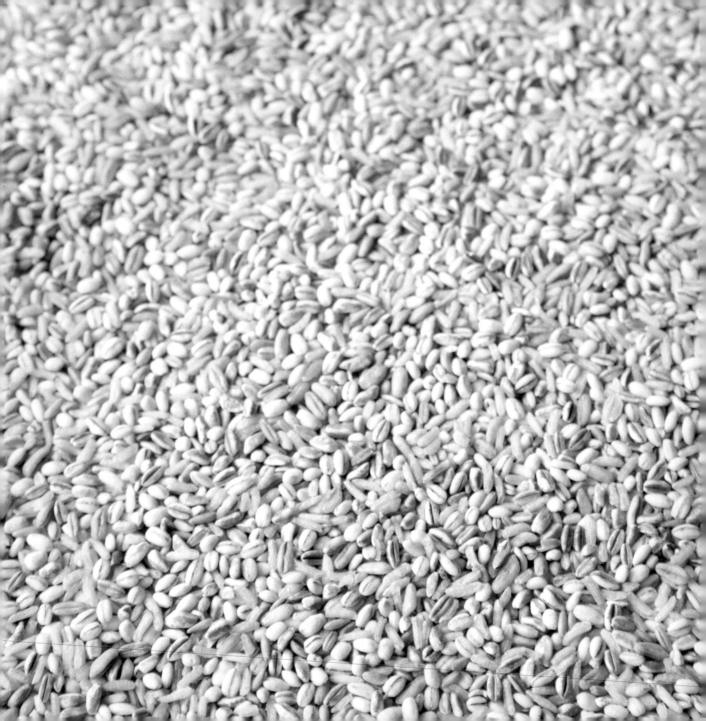